THIS BOOK BELONGS TO:

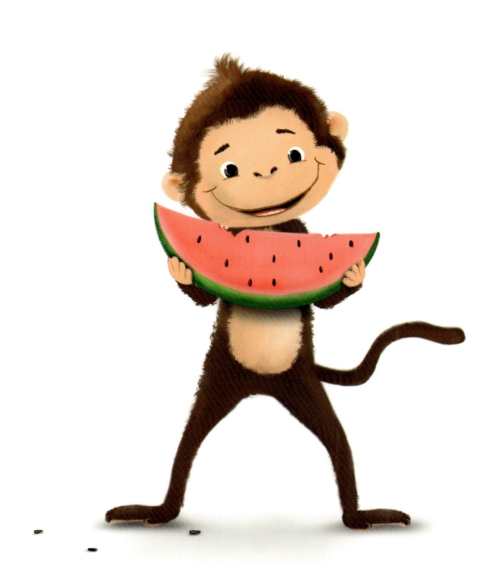

My Magical Foods

The Magic of Me Series

Copyright @ 2020 Becky Cummings

All rights reserved. No part of this publication may be reproduced, distributed, or transmitted in any form or by any means, including photocopying, recording, or other electronic or mechanical methods, without the prior permission of the publisher, except in the case of brief quotations embodied in critical reviews and certain other non-commercial uses permitted by copyright law. For permissions contact:

authorbcummings@gmail.com

ISBN: 978-1-951597-09-2 (hardcover)
ISBN: 978-1-951597-11-5 (paperback)
ISBN: 978-1-951597-10-8 (ebook)

Library of Congress Control Number: 2020909177

Illustrations by Zuzana Svobodová
Book design by Zuzana Svobodová, Maškrtáreň
Editing by Laura Boffa

First printing edition 2020.

Boundless Movement

Visit www.authorbcummings.com

The Magic of Me
MY MAGICAL FOODS

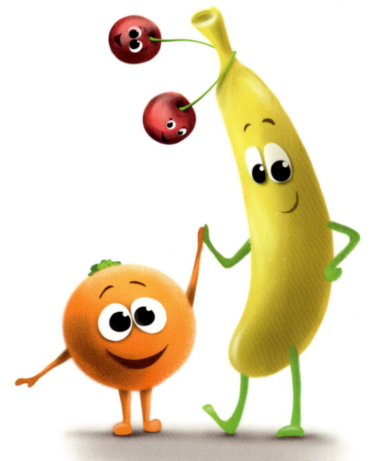

WRITTEN BY
BECKY CUMMINGS

ILLUSTRATED BY
ZUZANA SVOBODOVÁ

DEDICATION

To my niece and nephew, Maci and Landon.

The magic in you is bright! It shines through you to those you meet.

May you continue to feed your magic

and inspire the world!

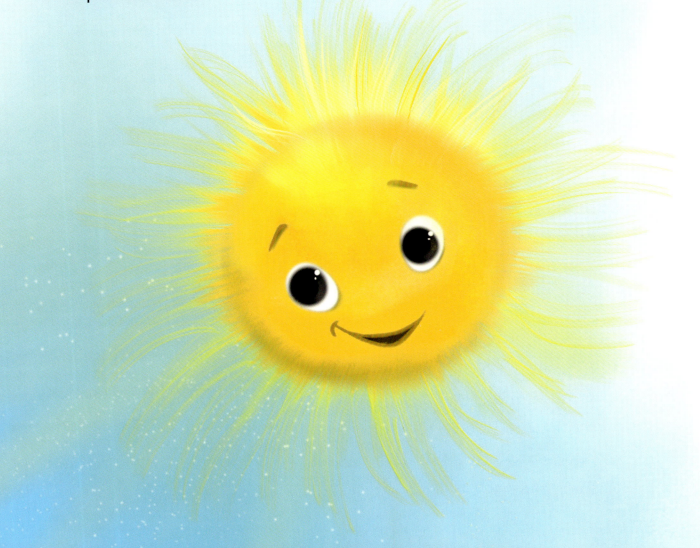

Tips for Teaching Children About Healthy Food Choices

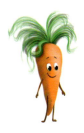

When grocery shopping with children, talk to them about best choices. Instead of labeling things as bad or good, which can lead to guilt or shame, use language to highlight the good qualities of a food or offer alternatives that are considered better choices. For example, if your child asks for potato chips, buy some potatoes instead and make homemade baked chips.

Involve your children when it comes to preparing meals or snacks. If they are older, they can even look up recipes. When children help gather ingredients, measure them, add them together and so on; it makes them more eager to try the final product. They will also understand what is inside their food.

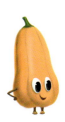

When introducing new foods or asking children to try foods they don't like, one thing you can try is the "One Bite Thank You Rule." This requires that they take one bite of anything on their plates and politely say, "Thank you." Children may be more open to trying new things if they know they only need to have one bite. After sampling a particular food on several occasions, kids may adjust to the flavor and enjoy a full serving.

The food that's best for you to eat,
are foods that grow below your feet!
In the dirt they have their birth.
They come to us from Mother Earth.

They'll make you grow up strong and smart.
So eat them now! Don't wait to start.
Open your mouth and enjoy the ride.
Feed your magic growing inside.

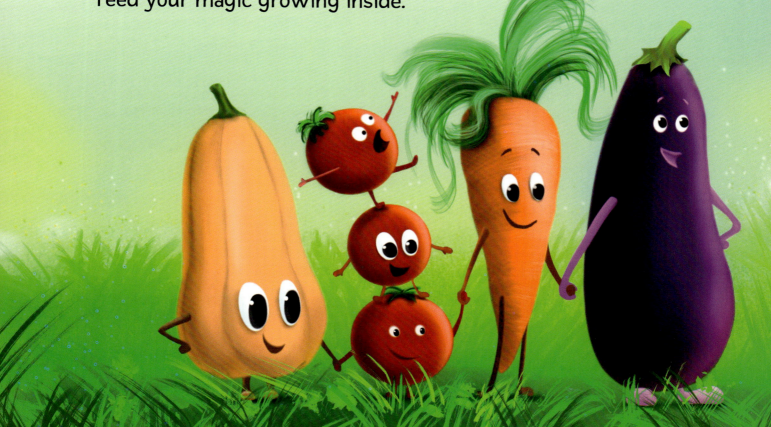

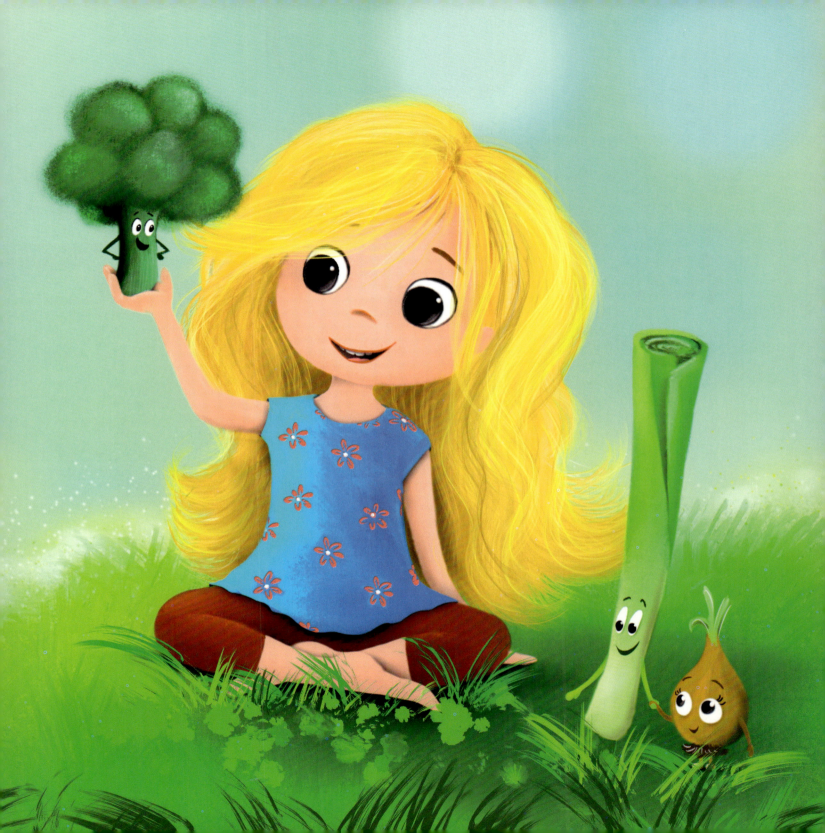

As tiny seeds these foods start small,

in time they'll grow up ripe and tall.

Oh, tiny seed, what will you be?

A PLANT,

   A FLOWER,

      OR A TREE.

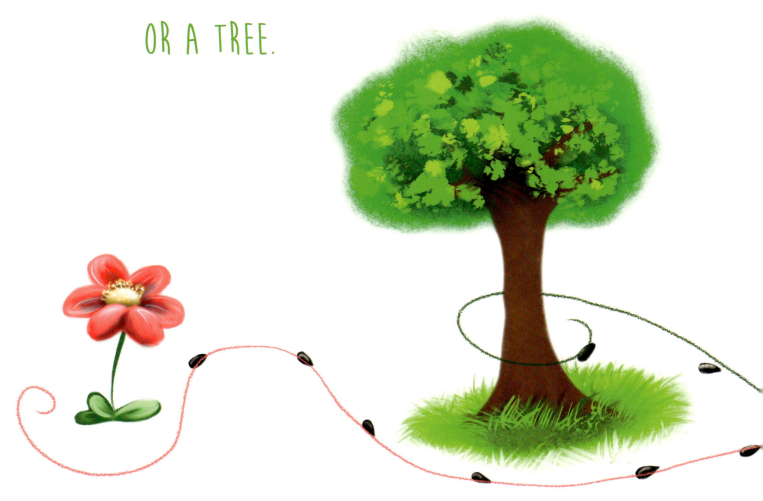

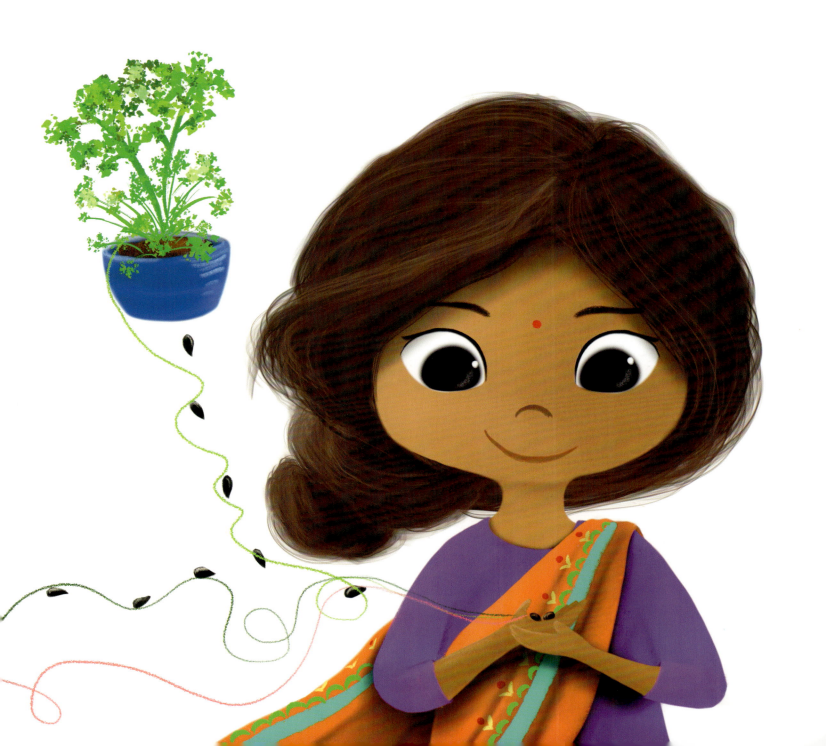

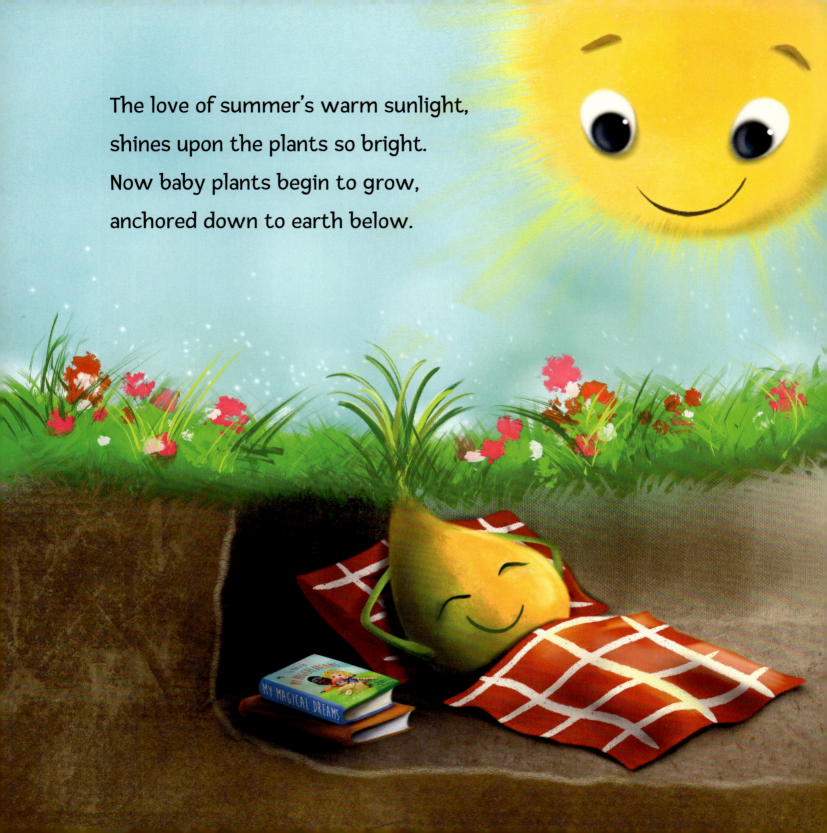

The love of summer's warm sunlight,
shines upon the plants so bright.
Now baby plants begin to grow,
anchored down to earth below.

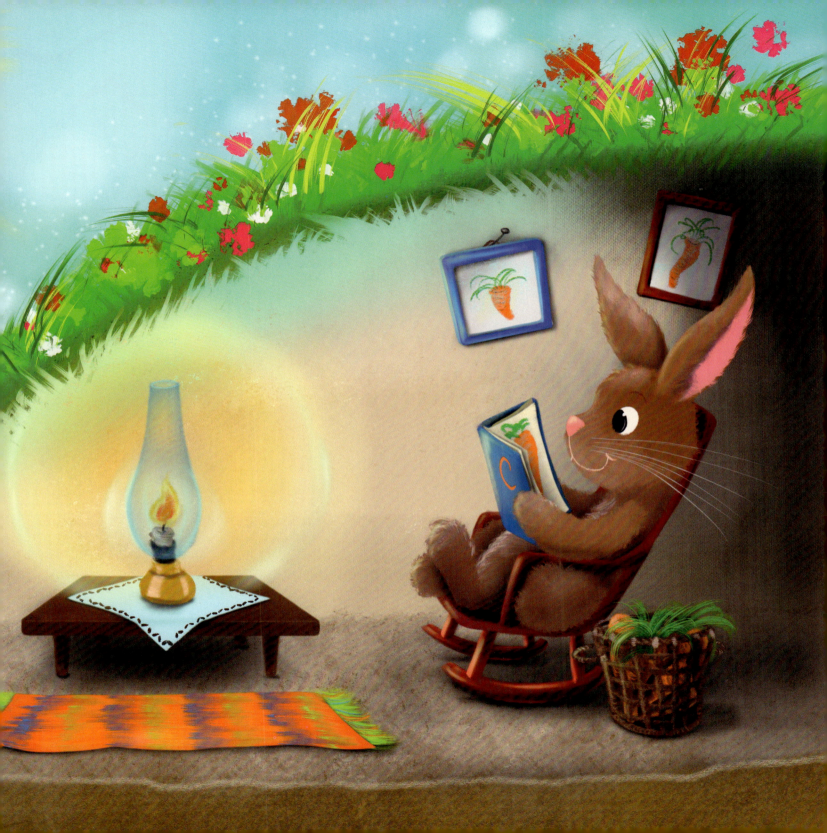

Up stems stretch, they rise so high.

Green leaves unfold to face the sky.

These leaves have sunlight for their lunch.

They sip in silence, without a crunch.

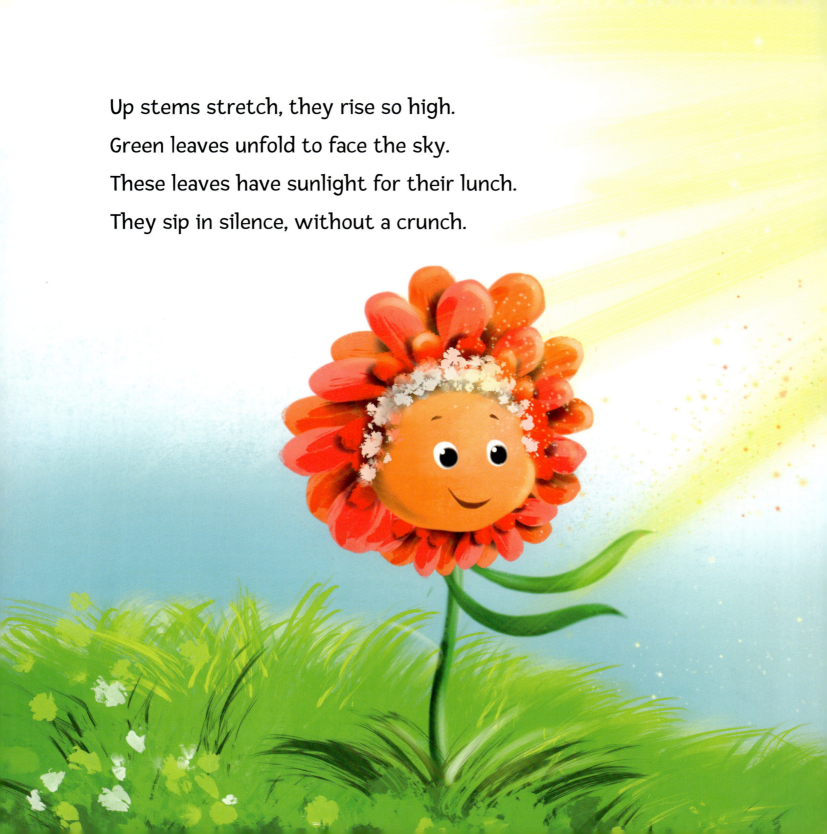

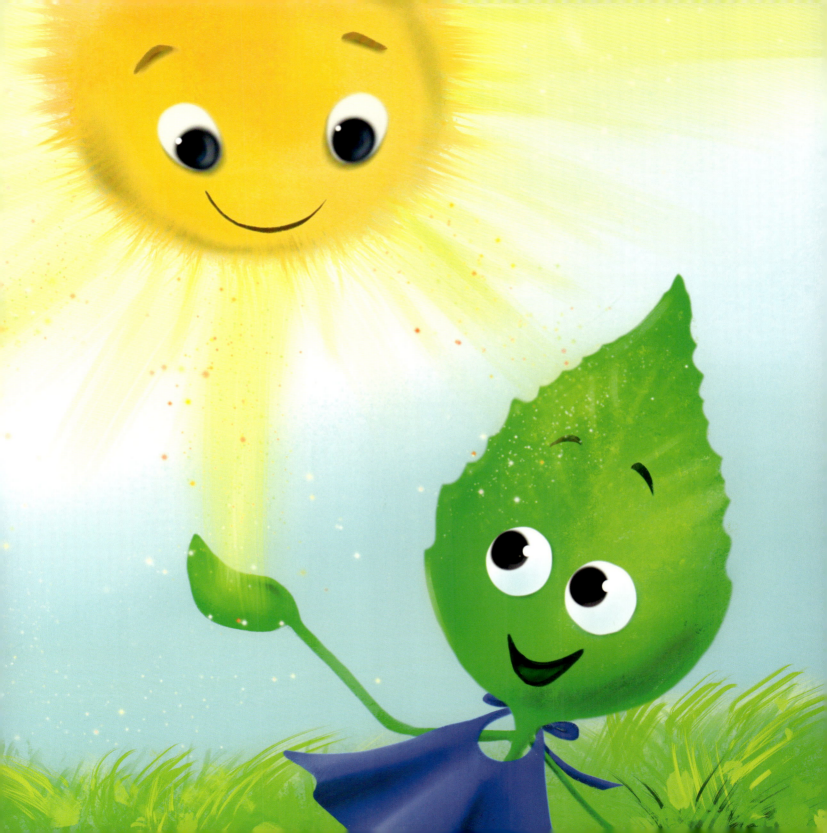

Strong roots drink water from the ground,
and pull in minerals from all around.
The plants will sprout some fruits to eat,
or leaves and veggies, what a treat!

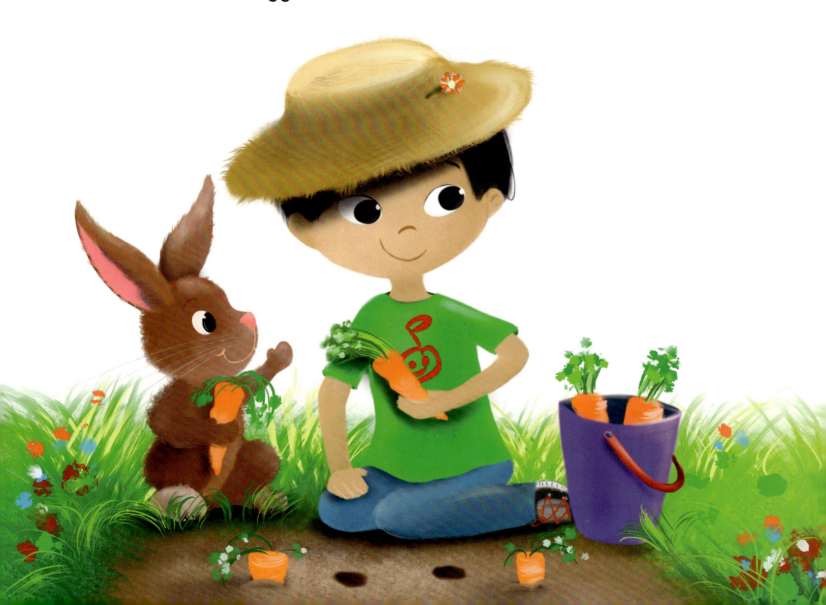

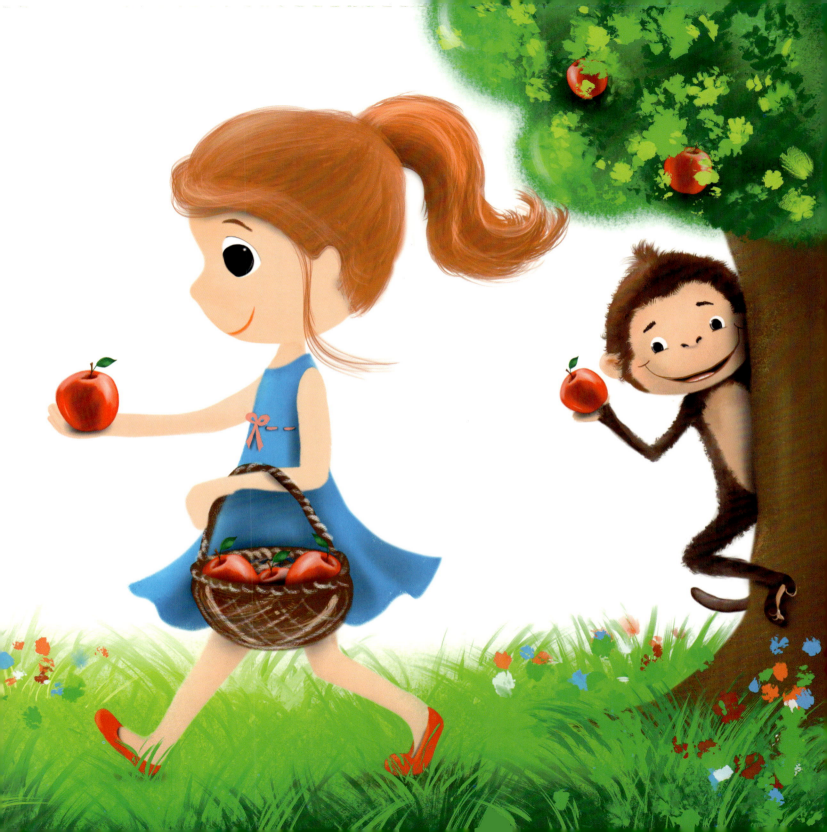

Animals can understand,
about the best food in the land.
Look how giraffes grow very tall,
by eating twigs and leaves,

THAT'S ALL!

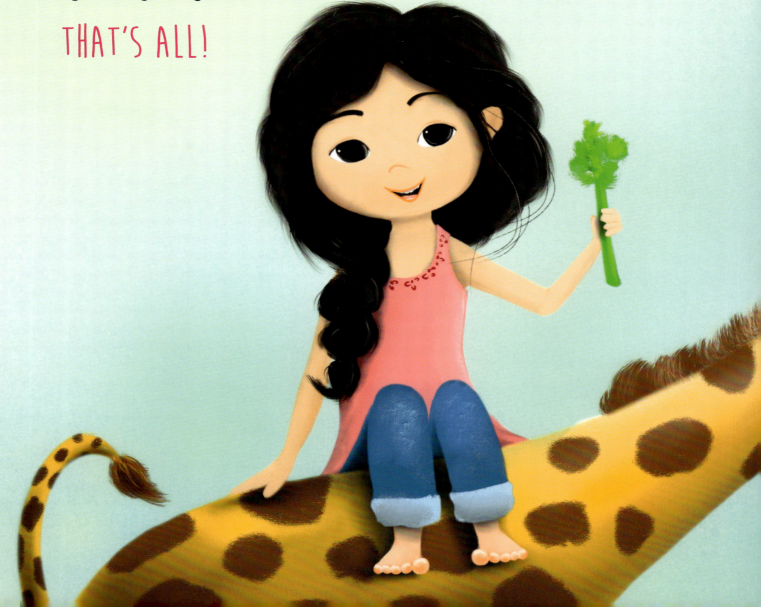

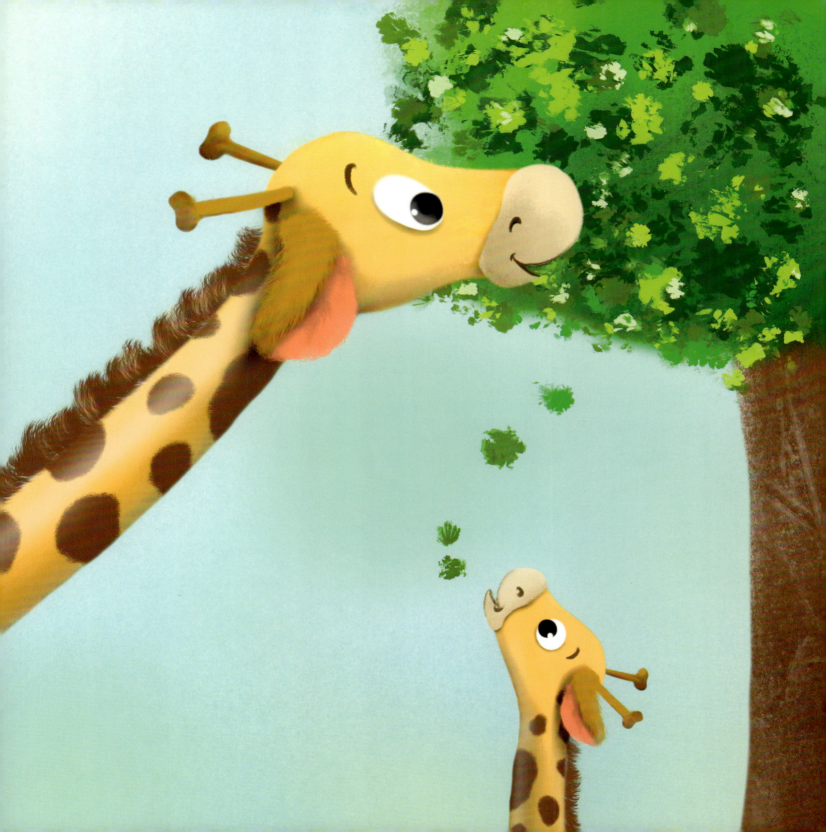

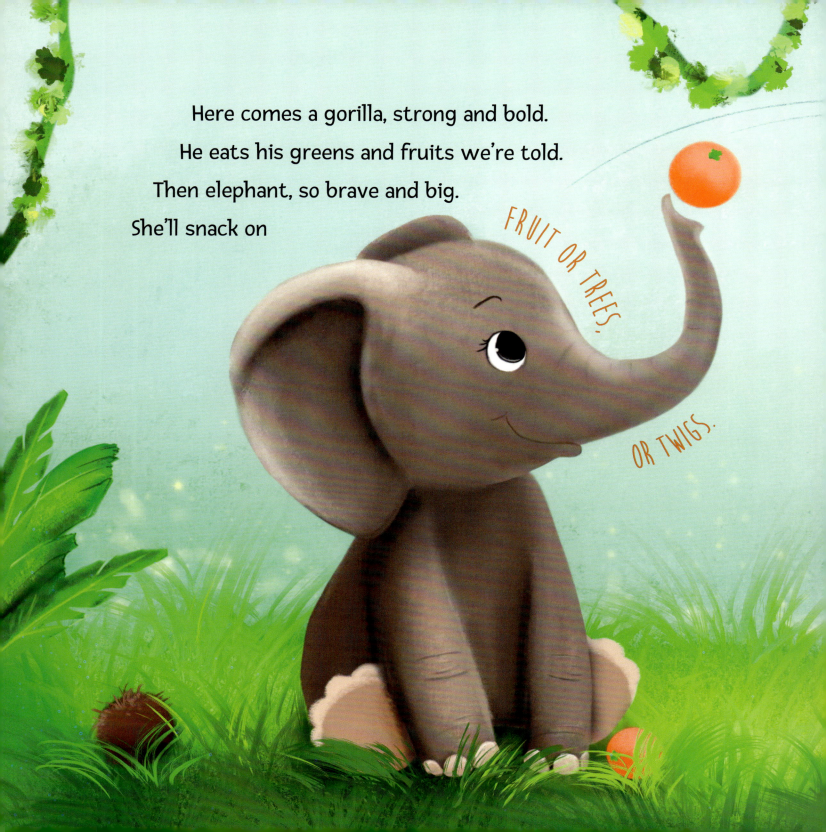

Here comes a gorilla, strong and bold.
He eats his greens and fruits we're told.
Then elephant, so brave and big.
She'll snack on FRUIT OR TREES, OR TWIGS.

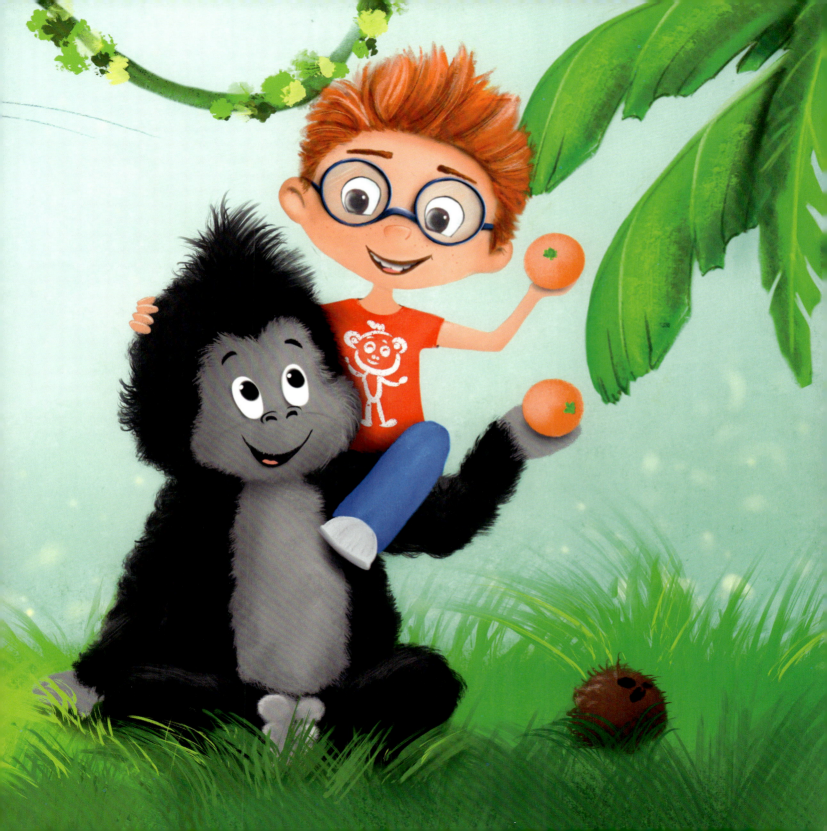

Now it's your turn to fuel on up.

In the morning start with a cup.

Lemon loves a big old squeeze,

in warm water, she says, "Please!"

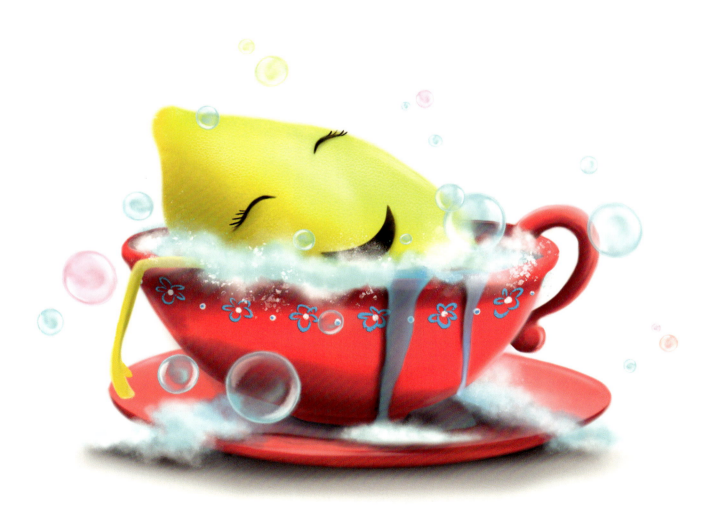

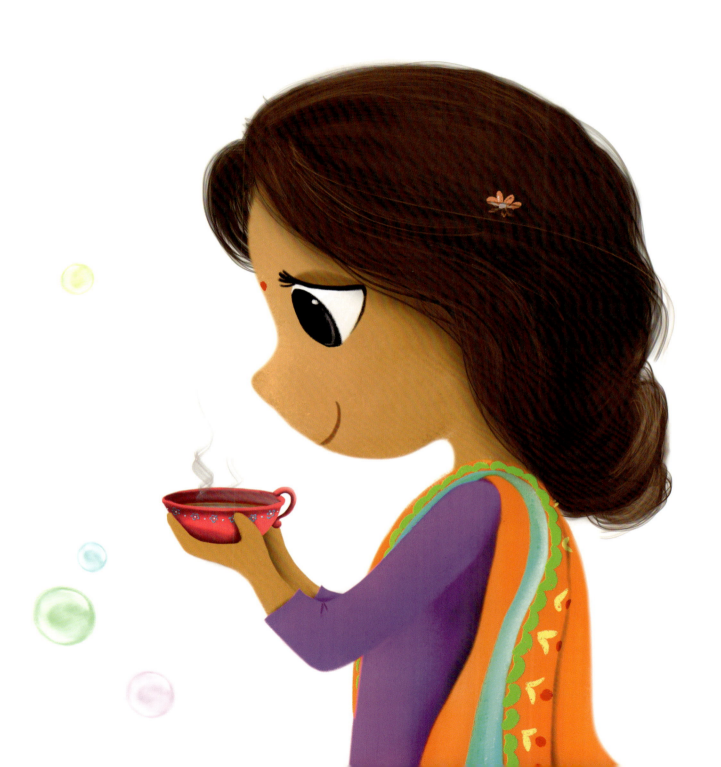

Mash avocado, she won't care.
Dip or spread her anywhere.
The spinach wants to join on in,

WITH MANGO IN A SMOOTHIE SPIN.

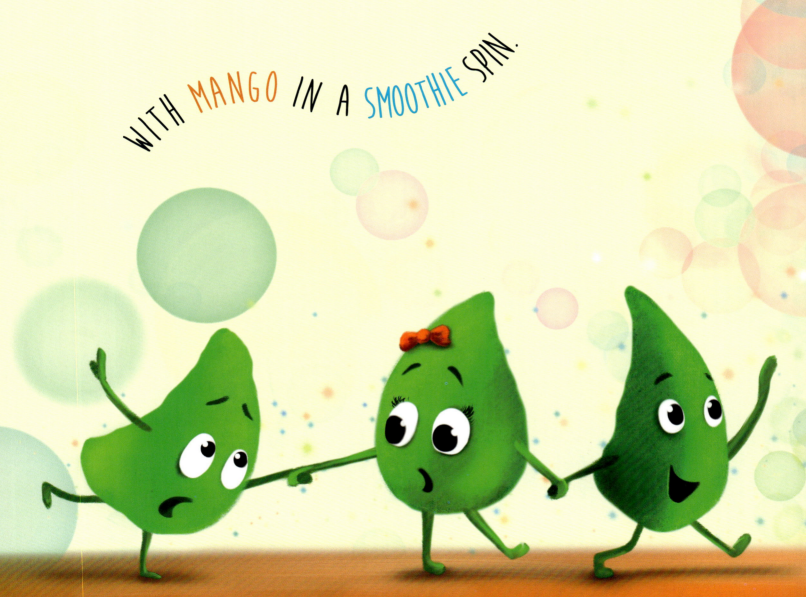

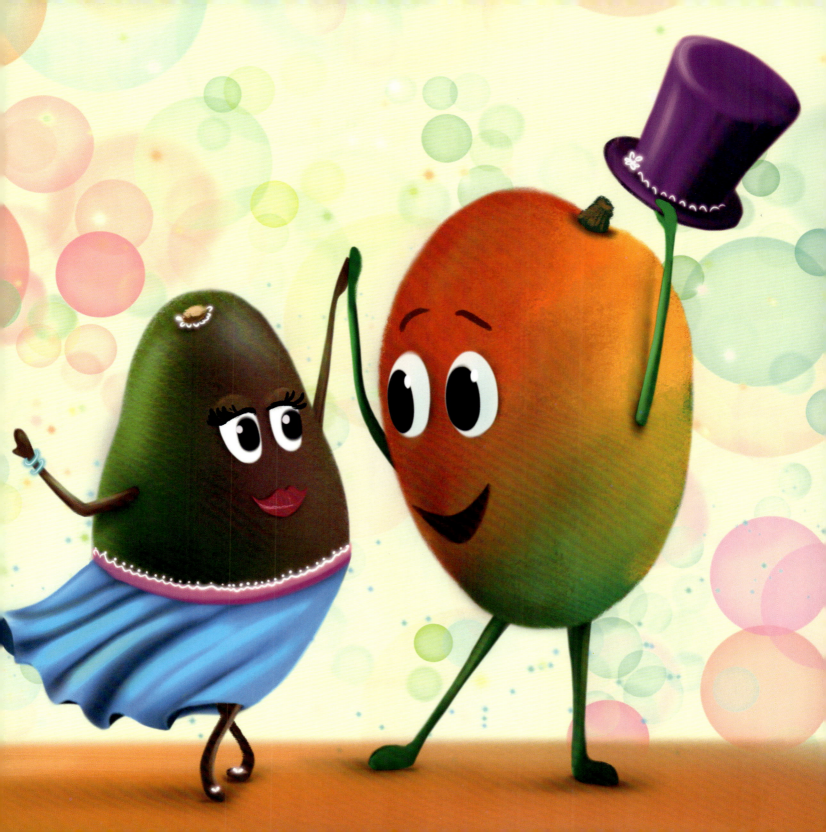

Ice pop bananas are a dream.

Or turn them into cold ice cream.

Top with berries, super bold.

These foods can help you fight a cold.

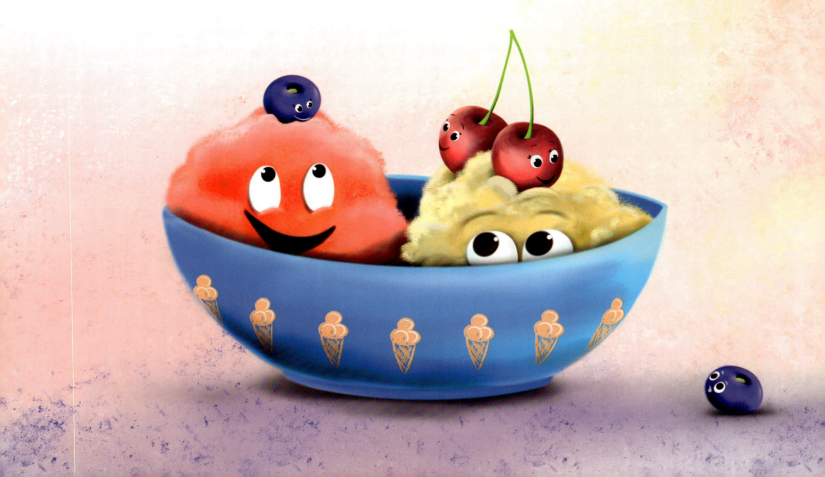

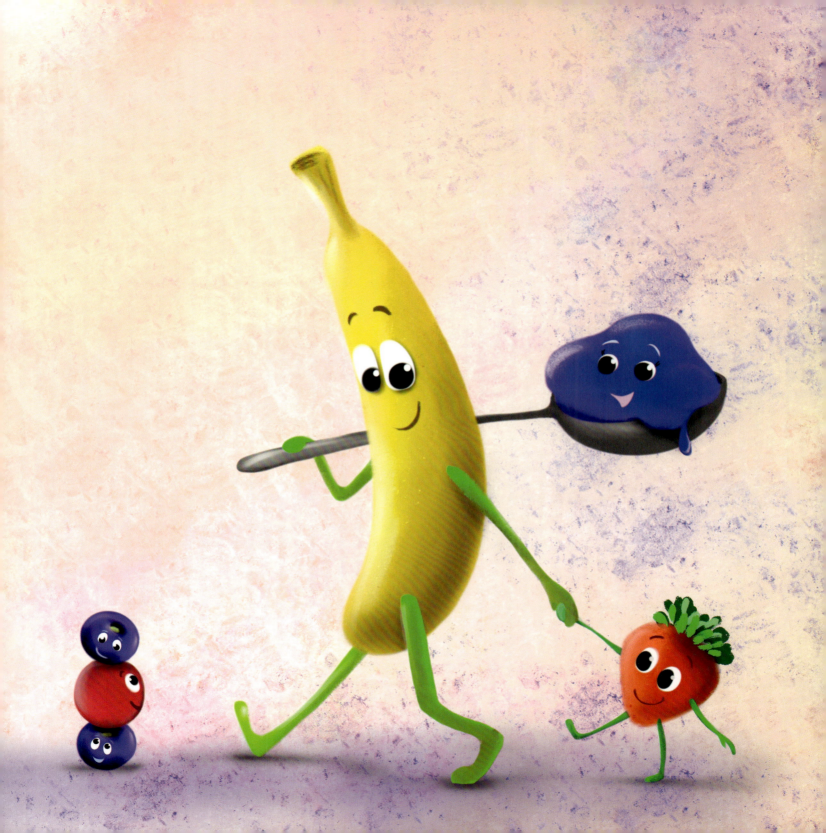

Let's make a list of foods to try.
Pick one to start, now don't be shy!
One bite, thank you, is a must.
Soon your taste buds will adjust.

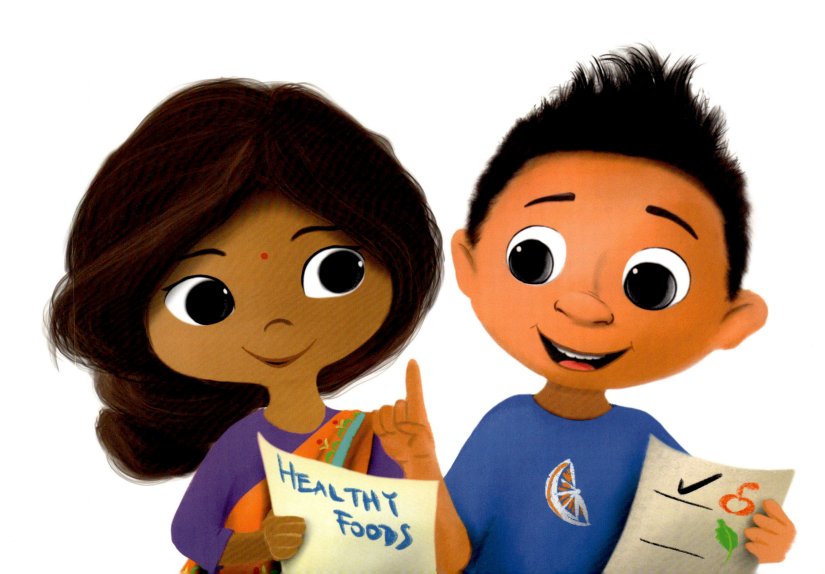

My List of Foods to Try

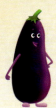
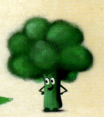

- ___ Carrot Sticks
- ___ Pepper Sticks
- ___ Cherry Tomatoes
- ___ Hummus with Veggies or Pita Bread
- ___ Unsweetened Applesauce
- ___ Bananas
- ___ Grapes
- ___ Blueberries
- ___ Strawberries
- ___ Apples
- ___ Raisins
- ___ Celery
- ___ Mild Salsa and Chips
- ___ Guacamole and Rice Cakes
- ___ Granola
- ___ Pumpkin Seeds
- ___ Watermelon
- ___ Peaches
- ___ Roasted Crunchy Chickpeas
- ___ Veggie Chips
- ___ Sliced Cucumbers
- ___ Edamame
- ___ Snap Peas
- ___ Pears
- ___ Clementines
- ___ Banana or Apple Chips
- ___ Air-Popped Popcorn
- ___ Sunflower Seeds

It's time for lunch, so don't be late.
Grab your fork, a spoon and plate!
Eat tons of fruits and veggies too.
Fill your belly! They're good for you.

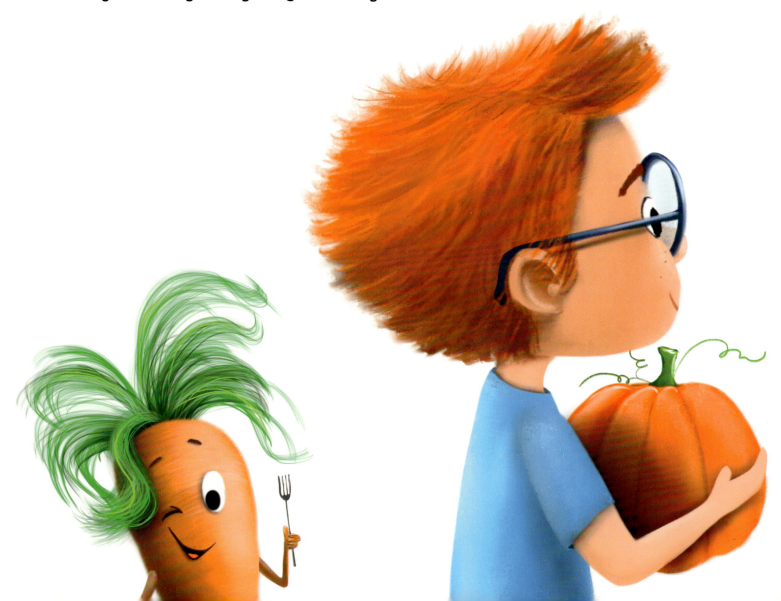

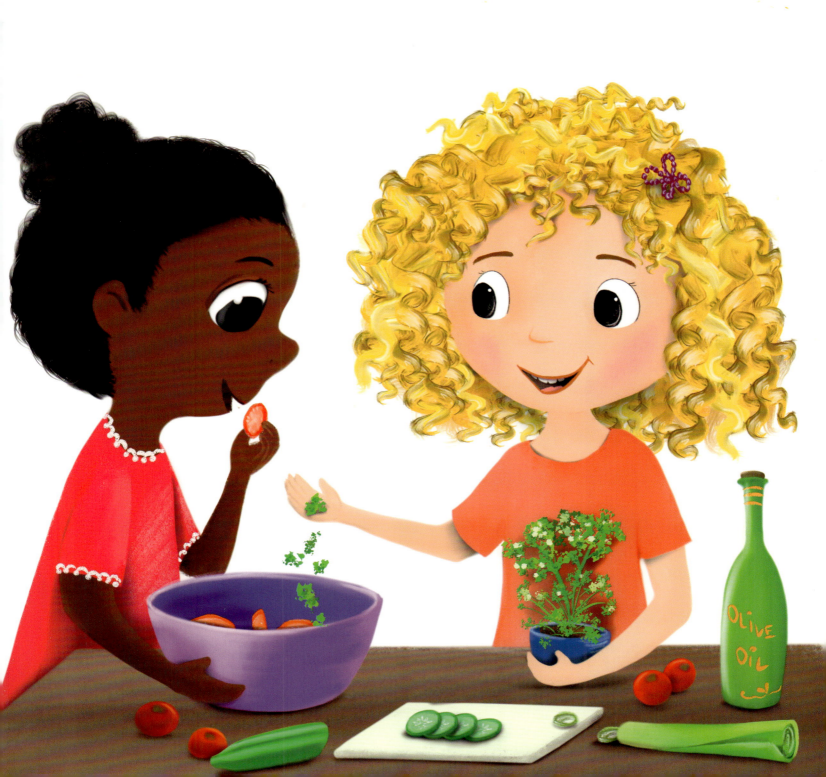

These foods have power to help you heal,
so make them part of every meal!
Your body needs fuel just like a car,
to spread your magic wide and far.

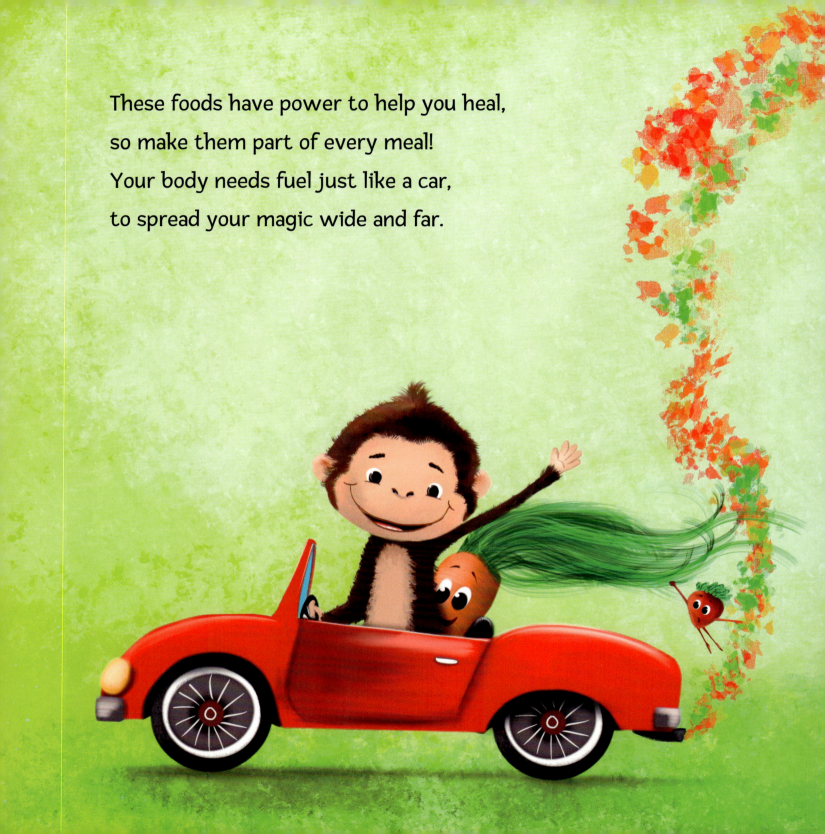

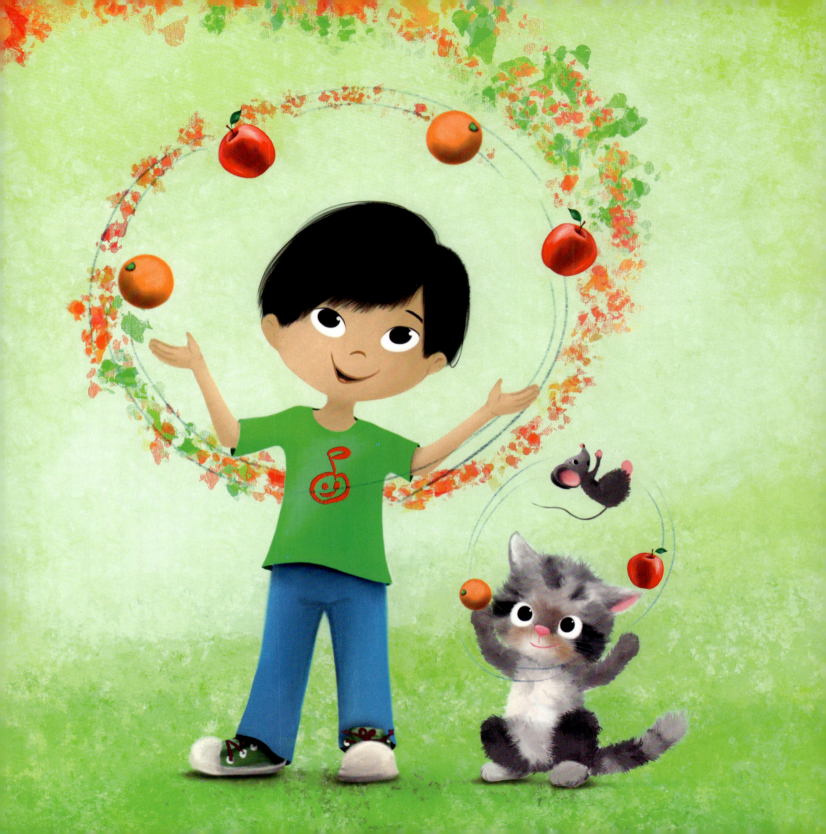

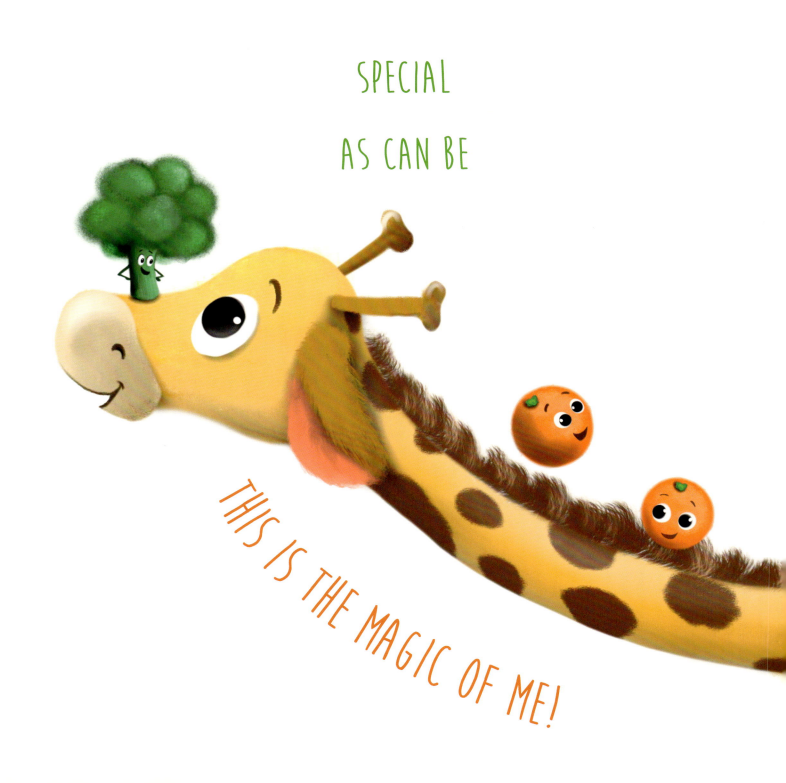

SPECIAL AS CAN BE

THIS IS THE MAGIC OF ME!

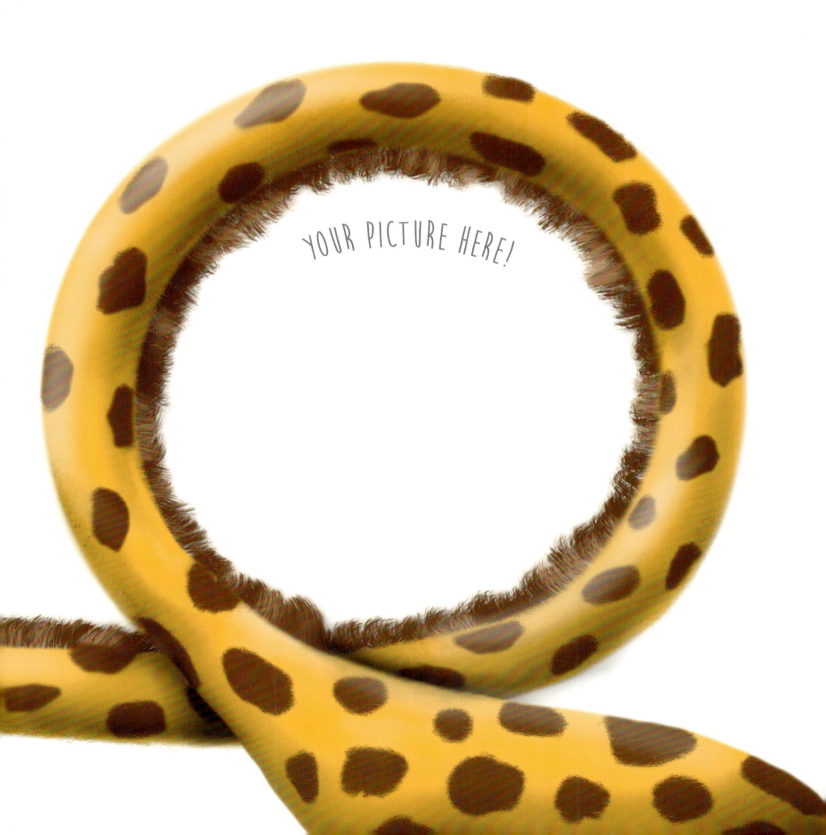

Dear Readers,

Thank you for reading *My Magical Foods* to your child or children. Healthy eating begins at home. Children are learning important habits that will last a lifetime, so now is the time to instill wisdom about food. Make it an enjoyable experience by involving your children when it comes to grocery shopping and preparing meals or snacks.

If you feel *My Magical Foods* should be shared with others, the best way to help it reach more children is to leave an honest review on Amazon and share it on social media. Your words and photos will help others learn about my book and encourage me to keep on writing!

If you enjoyed this book, be sure to check out my other books.

Your support is a blessing. Thank you!

With love,

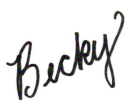

#themagicofme
@authorbcummings

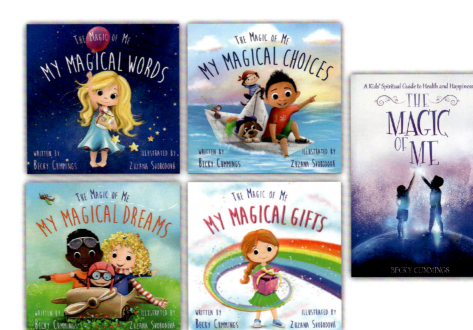

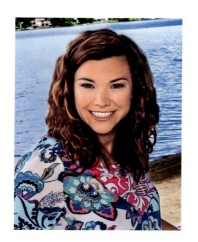

Becky Cummings is an author, teacher and mom of three. She loves kids and speaking her truth. Becky is blessed to combine these passions by writing children's books that spread messages of love, hope, faith, health, and happiness. When she isn't writing, you might find her salsa dancing, eating a veggie burrito at her favorite Mexican joint, or traveling to new places! Becky is available for author visits and wants to connect with you so be sure to visit her on Facebook fb.me/authorbcummings, or Instagram and visit her website, www.authorbcummings.com.

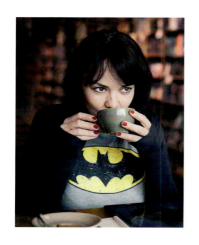

Zuzana Svobodová is an illustrator. She uses both digital and traditional techniques, as well as the world of fantasy delivered happily by her two children to bring stories to life. When she isn't working on illustrations, she enjoys drawing, doing and teaching yoga, dreaming and baking sweets.

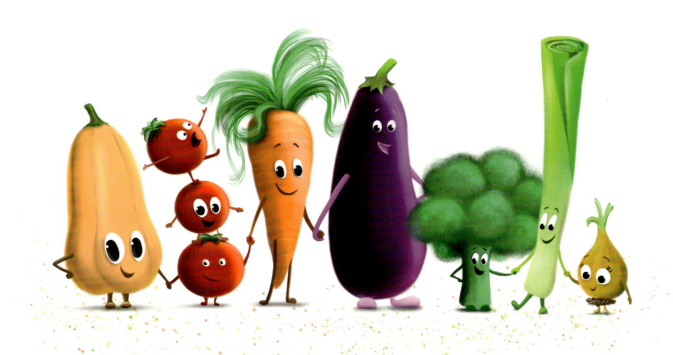